Superfoods Cookbook
[Second Edition]

Powerful Foods to Energize, Detoxify, and
Lead a Healthy Lifestyle

Sandra C. Anderson

Table of Contents

SUPERFOODS COOKBOOK..1

MAIN DISHES...6

Pinto Bean Tacos 6
BBQ-Style Salmon with Kale 8
Salmon with Lemon Butter Sauce.......................................10
Avocado and Black Bean Wraps...11
Brown Rice Bowl with Shrimp and Broccoli.............................12
Moroccan-Style Chicken with Quinoa 13
Cauliflower and Chickpea Curry.......................................15
Pasta with White Beans, Tomatoes and Basil 16
Sardine Sandwiches 17
Stuffed Tomatoes 18
Sesame Noodles with Vegetables 19
Chipotle Salmon with Peanut Salsa 21
Spinach and Cheese Bread Pudding.....................................23
Sweet Potato and Walnut Casserole....................................25
Stuffed Onions 27
Collard Greens with Bacon 29
Tomato and Cheese Tart 30
Spicy Corn and Sweet Potato Soup.....................................32
Easy Caramelized Onion Pizza 34
Roasted Squash & Kale Salad..36
Broiled Salmon with Green Beans 38
Kale and White Bean Stew 41
Baked Beets 43
Bean and Barley Vegetable Soup.......................................45
Chickpeas and Mustard Greens with a Balsamic Glaze...................47
Rigatoni with Walnuts, Italian Sausage and Broccoli Rabe.............49
Cabbage Rolls 52
Steak with Roast Vegetables 54
Spicy Beef Soup..56
Slow Cooker Beef and Sweet Potato Curry 58

SIDE DISHES AND APPETIZERS 60

Roasted Eggplant Salad 60

Pomegranate Carrots.. 63

Broccoli with Bell Peppers 64

Leeks with Vinaigrette... 66

Chickpea and Sweet Potato Dip..................................... 68

Quinoa Salad with Kale and Avocado 70

Pumpkin and Flax Seed Dip 71

Spinach Salad with Fruit and Almonds 73

Roasted Brussels Sprouts.. 74

Roasted Garlic Soup 75

Bagna Cauda.. 77

Red Bean Dip.. 78

Quinoa Salad with Lemon Vinaigrette 79

Cranberry Salsa... 81

BREAKFAST 82

Blueberry-Walnut Muffins 82

Oatmeal-Blueberry Pancakes.. 84

Apple – Flax Seed Muffins.. 86

An Apple a Day Smoothie 88

Apple Bran Muffins with Streusel 89

Apple Cinnamon Bread with Raisins.............................. 91

Apple Cinnamon Toast... 93

Baked Cranberry Oatmeal 95

Blackberry Smoothie 97

Blueberry Apple Pancakes 98

Cherry Oatmeal Bars 100

Energy Nut Bars 102

Granola Bars... 104

Apple Honey Muffins 105

Buttermilk Fruit Nut Muffins 107

California Blueberry Smoothie 109

Honey Bran Muffins... 110

Hot Quinoa Breakfast Cereal...................................... 112

Loose Granola... 113

Oatmeal Nut Bars 115

Oatmeal with Cinnamon Apples.................................. 117

Peach Berry Smoothie 118

Peanut Butter Muffins.. 119

Pumpkin Apple Smoothie... 121

DESSERTS AND SNACKS 122

Roasted Nuts 122
Granola Bars with Fruit...124
Blueberry Shortbread Bars...126
Blueberry, Chocolate and Walnut Parfait.......................................128
Dark Chocolate Cake 129

SUPERFOODS COOKBOOK CONCLUSION 131

Superfoods Cookbook

It would be wonderful to make the claim that eating the Super Food diet would keep you from getting sick. Perhaps it is not too farfetched to say such a thing since it is the nutrients in the super foods that help to strengthen the immune system, which is what fights off illnesses and infections.

People on this diet can accurately make this claim though. People even claim to be cured of simple ailments like allergies when they changed their diets to super foods. While claims are made, it is truly an individual thing. While we cannot make this claim for sure, we can say that by consuming super foods you are giving your body the best chances at never being sick.

One of the biggest benefits to strengthening the immune system is also a metabolism booster, which gives you the energy to get up and move. Dieting is effective by itself, but it is more effective if done in conjunction with routine exercise too. Eating the highly nutritious foods of the super food diet gives you enough energy to change your physical activities and to be able to get up and do what you need to do to keep the body is good physical shape.

It is when people become sedentary that illnesses take hold. Perhaps when people consume the wrong foods they are left more lethargic and are unable to have enough energy to get up and move about. If you fill the body with nutrients that both strengthen the immune system and boost the metabolism, you will feel inclined to do something to burn off the energy. The body is then able to release good substances in the form of "endorphins" during exercise. This is the body's way to produce a natural high and this only occurs if the body is healthy.

If you are just starting out on the super food diet try to incorporate some exercise into your routine. You can start small and work up to it. Sometimes at first, it is a matter of mind over will. You may not feel like getting up and moving, but often if you take that first step you will find it gets easier fast so start slow and small. Do low impact aerobics or something as simple as a walk. Just thirty minutes three times a week will start the momentum. Be sure to do a warm up to prepare the muscles for it and a cool down. Keep at it for the best chances at good health.

What are Superfoods?

As the saying goes, we are what we eat and people are becoming ever more conscious that this is the case – and that they'd rather not be consuming a long list of chemical additives which they probably can't even pronounce, much less identify as food! It's well known that diet is one of the keys to better health and simply put, some foods are better for you than others.

That's where superfoods come in. These are foods which offer a wealth of nutrients as well as antioxidants and other naturally occurring compounds which promote better health and even reduce the risk of many illnesses from minor to life threatening. Superfoods include a fairly wide variety of different fruits and vegetables; and to be perfectly honest, most of them are foods that you probably already knew were good for you.

In this cookbook, we've included recipes which incorporate many of the foods which are well known as the most nutritious, healthy dietary choices. We've also steered clear of the trends; as you're probably aware if you spend any time at all following the latest news about nutrition and fitness, it seems that there's a new "superfood" being trumpeted as the best thing ever almost every week, soon to be replaced by the next flavor of the month.

Not that many of these foods aren't healthy and certainly, there's nothing wrong with including some Spirulina or acai berries in your diet. Instead, we've decided to focus on superfoods which are, by and large, available at your average well-stocked supermarket.

One thing that you'll probably notice as you read and cook the recipes in this book is that many of the recipes here are vegetarian. Many nutritionists have long said that a diet which is largely vegetarian is better for you, although there is some difference of opinion on this subject as well.

However, the superfoods are all plant-based and they're the star of these recipes; many of these recipes are also flexible enough to add meat to them if you'd like to increase your protein intake. There is one exception to this rule: salmon, which you will find plenty of recipes for in this book. Basically, as long as you make sure to include plenty of the superfoods which take center stage in these recipes, you can fine tune the recipes to match your own tastes.

What Superfoods Should You Add To Your Diet?
As we've discussed above, many of the most nutritious

and healthiest foods are ones you probably already knew that you should be eating regularly. Sweet potatoes, salmon, kale and other dark leafy greens, garlic and onions, blueberries and other berries, tomatoes, beans, nuts and seeds are all superfoods which provide your body with the vitamins, minerals, fiber, antioxidants and omega-3 fatty acids it needs for optimal health. Along with whole grains and other healthy choices, a diet rich in superfoods like the ones used in these recipes can help you to live a longer, healthier and yes, even a happier life! Here's to your health!

Main Dishes

Pinto Bean Tacos

Number of servings: 1

Ingredients:

1 cup cooked (fresh or canned) pinto beans, drained and rinsed
4 whole grain tortillas
1 cup diced tomatoes
1 cup shredded lettuce (preferably Romaine)
¼ cup green onions, sliced
½ avocado, sliced
½ tsp cumin
1 tsp chili powder
Juice of 2 limes
Salsa, your choice

Preparation:

Mix together the pinto beans, lime juice, chili powder and cumin in a small saucepan (or microwave-safe bowl, if you'd prefer to microwave the beans) and warm through. While the beans are warming, toast the tortillas over the flame of a gas stove or microwave to warm and soften.

Divide the bean mixture among the tortillas and top with the diced tomatoes, chopped lettuce, avocado, green onions and salsa. Serve immediately.

BBQ-Style Salmon with Kale

Number of servings: 4

Ingredients:

4 salmon filets (about 4 ounces each)
4 tbsp barbecue sauce, your choice
2 cloves of garlic, minced
3 cups kale, roughly chopped
4 tsp olive oil
salt and black pepper, to taste

Preparation:

Brush the salmon filets with 2 tsp of the olive oil and barbecue sauce and place under the broiler. Cook for 8 minutes for each inch of thickness – remember that they'll continue to cook for a few minutes even after you remove them from the oven, so don't overdo it. If they're slightly undercooked, just put them back under the broiler for a minute – but if they end up being overcooked, there's nothing you can do about it.

While the salmon filets are cooking, sauté the garlic and kale in the remaining 2 tsp of olive oil over medium-high heat, stirring regularly. Cook until the garlic is fragrant and the kale is just wilted. Season to taste with salt and black pepper and divide the kale among four plates and top with the salmon filets. Serve immediately.

Salmon with Lemon Butter Sauce

Number of Servings: 4

Ingredients:

4 salmon filets, about 4 ounces each
4 tbsp butter
1 cup vegetable broth
Juice and zest of 2 lemons
2 cloves of garlic, crushed
2 tsp olive oil
salt and black pepper, to taste

Preparation:

Brush the salmon filets with olive oil and place under the broiler, cooking for 8 minutes for each inch of thickness. While the salmon filets cook, melt the butter in a medium saucepan and whisk in the lemon juice and zest, vegetable broth and crushed garlic. Bring to a simmer, stirring occasionally to prevent separation. Once the salmon filets are cooked, transfer to individual plates and drizzle with the lemon butter sauce, season to taste with salt and black pepper and serve hot.

Avocado and Black Bean Wraps

Number of servings: 4
1 cup black beans, canned or homemade, drained and
rinsed
4 whole grain tortillas
½ avocado, sliced
1 tsp cumin
1 tsp chili powder
juice of 1 lime
salsa (your choice)
diced onion and chopped cilantro, optional

Preparation:

Mix together the black beans, cumin, chili powder and
lime juice and warm in a small saucepan over medium
heat or in the microwave. While the bean mixture is
warming, toast the tortillas over the flame of a gas stove
or microwave to warm and soften. Divide the black bean
mixture among the four tortillas and top with the sliced
avocado, a little salsa and onion and cilantro, if using.
Fold up and serve immediately.

Brown Rice Bowl with Shrimp and Broccoli

Number of servings: 4

Ingredients:

12 large shrimp, cleaned, deveined and cooked
1 ½ cups broccoli florets
4 cloves of garlic, minced
1 cup brown rice, cooked
1 tbsp peanut oil
2 tbsp peanuts, finely chopped
soy sauce, to taste

Preparation:

Heat the peanut oil in a large skillet. Once the oil is hot, sauté the garlic for about 2 minutes, stirring occasionally. Add the broccoli florets and cook for another 5 – 8 minutes, stirring regularly until the broccoli is crisp-tender. Add the rice and shrimp and cook for another 4 – 5 minutes or until all ingredients are heated through. Season to taste with soy sauce, divide among four individual bowls and serve hot, topped with chopped peanuts.

Moroccan-Style Chicken with Quinoa

Number of servings: 6

Ingredients:

1 lb. chicken breast, boneless and skinless, cooked
1 cup water
½ cup dry quinoa
juice of 2 lemons
1 tbsp olive oil (use extra virgin olive oil)
1 tsp cumin
½ tsp cinnamon
2 tbsp raisins
2 tbsp fresh mint, chopped
salt and black pepper, to taste
lemon wedges, for garnish

Preparation:

Bring 1 cup water and ½ cup quinoa to a boil in a small saucepan; reduce to a simmer and cook, covered for 10 – 15 minutes, or until all of the water has been absorbed. Reheat the chicken breast and divide into four roughly equal servings. Fluff the quinoa with a fork and add the mint, lemon juice, olive oil and raisins. Stir well to combine and season to taste with salt and black pepper. Divide the quinoa among four individual plates, top with the chicken breast and serve with lemon wedges on the side.

Cauliflower and Chickpea Curry

Number of servings: 4 (6 if served as a side dish)

Ingredients:

1 ½ cups cauliflower, chopped
½ cup cooked chickpeas, canned or homemade, drained and rinsed
1 cup cooked brown rice
1 small white or yellow onion, diced
2 tbsp raisins
1 tbsp vegetable oil
2 tsp curry powder (or more to taste)
1 – 2 green onions, sliced
salt, to taste

Preparation:

Heat the vegetable oil in a large skillet or saucepan. Once the oil is hot, add the onion and sauté for 2-3 minutes or until it starts to turn translucent. Add the curry powder and cook for another 1-2 minutes, stirring occasionally. Next, add the chickpeas, raisins and green onions and cook for 3 – 5 minutes or until all ingredients are heated through. Season to taste with salt and curry powder and serve over the cooked brown rice.

Pasta with White Beans, Tomatoes and Basil

Number of servings: 4

Ingredients:

1 cup cooked white beans (cannellini, etc.), drained and
rinsed
½ cup dry whole grain penne or fusilli
1 cup halved cherry tomatoes (diced Roma tomatoes
may be substituted)
3 tbsp roughly chopped fresh basil
1 clove of garlic, crushed
2 tbsp balsamic vinegar or red wine vinegar
2 tbsp Parmesan or Romano cheese, grated
1 tbsp olive oil (use extra virgin olive oil if possible)
Salt and black pepper, to taste

Preparation:

Cook the whole grain pasta as per the directions on the
package and toss with the white beans, chopped basil,
tomatoes, crushed garlic, olive oil and vinegar. Season to
taste with salt and black pepper and serve topped with
grated Parmesan or Romano cheese.

Sardine Sandwiches

Number of servings: 4

Ingredients:

2 cans sardines in olive oil
8 slices of whole grain bread, toasted
2 tbsp pickles (your choice), drained and finely chopped
1 tbsp minced red onion
2 tbsp mayonnaise
1 tomato, thinly sliced
1 avocado, sliced
2 cups arugula or spinach
Salt and black pepper, to taste

Preparation:

Drain the sardines and place in a small bowl, along with the mayonnaise, minced red onion and chopped pickles. Mix well to combine and season to taste with salt and black pepper. Divide the sardine mixture among four slices of bread and top with tomato slices, arugula or spinach leaves and avocado slices before adding another slice of bread and serving.

Stuffed Tomatoes

Number of servings: 8

Ingredients:

8 medium-sized tomatoes
2 ½ cups cooked brown rice
1 cup toasted pine nuts
1 cup chopped fresh basil
1/3 cup olive oil
salt and black pepper, to taste

Preparation:

Start by preheating your oven to 400 F. Slice the tops off of each tomato and scoop out most of the flesh (a grapefruit spoon works well for this). Mix together the brown rice, pine nuts, basil and olive oil and season to taste with salt and black pepper. Fill each tomato with the rice and pine nut mixture. Place the tomatoes on a lightly oiled baking sheet and bake for 20 minutes. Serve hot or cool and serve at room temperature.

Sesame Noodles with Vegetables

Number of servings: 4

Ingredients:

4 cups cooked soba (Japanese buckwheat noodles) –
about 6 oz. uncooked*
4 cups baby spinach
1 cup shelled Edamame (green soybeans)
2/3 cup of strong, freshly brewed green tea
2 tbsp toasted sesame oil
3 cloves of garlic, minced
1" inch long piece of fresh ginger, peeled and minced or
crushed
2 medium size zucchini or yellow crookneck squash,
halved lengthwise and sliced about ¼" thick
2 tsp sesame seeds
juice and zest of 1 lemon
soy sauce, to taste
* whole grain fettuccine may be substituted if you can't
find soba noodles

Preparation:

Heat 1 tbsp of sesame oil in a large skillet and sauté the
garlic for about 1 minute, then add the ginger and cook

for another minute. Add the sliced zucchini or yellow squash and sauté for another 3 minutes, until the zucchini is crisp-tender. Add the green tea, Edamame and a splash of soy sauce and bring to a simmer, then add the spinach, lemon juice and zest, the sesame seeds and the remaining 1 tbsp of sesame oil, stir once and remove from heat.

Serve the vegetable mixture over the cooked noodles, reserving any remaining cooking liquid to serve on the side.

Chipotle Salmon with Peanut Salsa

Number of servings: 8

Ingredients:

8 salmon fillets, about 4 – 5 ounces each
8 cloves of garlic
5 chipotle peppers in adobo sauce
2 cups roasted peanuts, salted or unsalted
2 dried ancho or guajillo chilies, stemmed, seeded and
chopped
½ cup honey
juice of 2 limes
salt, to taste
a little chopped cilantro, for garnish

Preparation:

For the salsa:
Roast the garlic cloves in a dry skillet over medium heat
for about 15 minutes, turning occasionally until the
garlic is softened and begins to blacken. Remove from
heat and set aside the garlic to cool – peel the garlic
once it has cooled.

While the garlic cools, toast the ancho or guajillo

peppers in the same skillet until aromatic (this should take 3 -5 minutes). Place the toasted chilies in a bowl and cover with hot water. Allow the peppers to rehydrate for about 30 minutes. Drain the peppers and transfer to a food processor along with the toasted garlic, the peanuts and 3 of the chipotle peppers. Add just a little bit of lime juice and blend until smooth, adding more juice if needed. Season to taste with salt and transfer to a bowl.

For the salmon:
Heat your oven to broil. While the oven heats, add the honey, a pinch of salt and the remaining 2 chipotle peppers. Process until the ingredients form a smooth puree.

Broil the salmon filets on a lightly oiled baking sheet for 2 minutes per side. Remove from the broiler and brush with the chipotle-honey glaze. Broil for another 2 minutes or until the salmon reaches your desired level of doneness. Serve hot with peanut salsa and garnished with chopped cilantro.

Spinach and Cheese Bread Pudding

Number of servings: 6

Ingredients:

8 thick slices of whole grain bread, cut into 1" cubes
1 10 ounce package of frozen spinach, thawed and drained
6 large eggs
2 cups milk (whole or 2%, not skim)
1 cup shredded cheese (sharp cheddar works well, but any cheese you like will do fine)
1 tsp nutmeg
1 tsp dried thyme
salt and black pepper, to taste

Preparation:

Start by preheating your oven to 375 F. While the oven is heating, beat the eggs, milk, thyme, nutmeg and a pinch each of salt and black pepper (or more, if desired) with a whisk until well blended. Fold in the spinach, shredded cheese and bread cubes.

Lightly oil a large glass or ceramic baking dish and pour in the mixture. Bake until the bread pudding puffs up and browns on top, about 25 minutes. You can tell if the pudding is done when a knife inserted into the center comes out clean. Once the bread pudding is finished, remove from the oven and allow it to stand for 5 – 10 minutes to set before slicing and serving.

Sweet Potato and Walnut Casserole

Number of servings: 8

Ingredients:

5 large sweet potatoes, cut into ¾" thick slices
½ cup coarsely chopped walnuts
4 tbsp butter, cut into small pieces
2 tbsp dark brown sugar
Salt and black pepper, to taste

Preparation:

Preheat your oven to 400 F. Arrange half of the sliced sweet potatoes to form a single layer in a large glass or ceramic baking dish. Sprinkle the layer of sweet potatoes with 1 tbsp of the brown sugar, half of the butter pieces, a little salt and plenty of black pepper. Repeat the process with the remaining sweet potatoes and butter, brown sugar, salt and pepper.

Cover the dish with foil and bake for 30 minutes. Remove the foil and top the casserole with walnuts and bake for another 40 minutes, uncovered or until the sweet potatoes are tender. Baste the casserole with the syrup formed in the dish every ten minutes while you're baking it uncovered. Once the casserole is finished, remove from heat, allow it to stand for 5 minutes and serve.

Stuffed Onions

Number of servings:

Ingredients:

4 large yellow onions
2 lbs. parsnips, peeled (optional) and sliced into 1/2"
thick rounds
1 cup chicken or vegetable broth
½ cup crumbled Roquefort cheese
¼ cup walnuts, toasted and chopped
1 tbsp butter
½ tbsp olive oil
1 tsp salt
1 tsp black pepper, or to taste

Preparation:

Preheat your oven to 425 F. While it heats, melt the butter in a medium saucepan and add the sliced parsnips, salt and pepper. Cook over medium heat for 5 minutes, add the broth and cook, covered, for about 15 minutes or until the parsnips are tender. Allow the parsnips to cool for about 10 minutes and transfer the parsnips and broth to a food processor; blend until it becomes a smooth puree. Set the puree aside.

The next step is to roast the onions. Line a large baking pan with foil. Slice a thin slice from the bottom of each onion to prevent them from rolling and cut about half an inch off of the top of each onion. Using a small knife, cut out most of the inside of the onion, leaving a few layers (about half an inch) on the outside. Chop the centers of the onions finely and mix into the pureed parsnips. Stuff each onion with the mixture, rub with olive oil and place on the foil covered baking pan.

Bake for 1 ½ hours, top the onions with Roquefort and walnut and return to the oven for another 5 – 10 minutes. Remove from the oven and serve at once.

Collard Greens with Bacon

Number of servings: 8

Ingredients:

2 large bunches of collard greens, washed, patted dry
and cut into ¾" strips
½ lb. thick cut bacon, cooked and crumbled
4 cloves of garlic, crushed
¼ cup olive oil
2 tbsp whole grain brown mustard
2 tbsp apple cider vinegar
salt and black pepper, to taste

Preparation:

Mix together 3 tbsp of the olive oil, the mustard, vinegar
and a little salt and pepper in a small bowl. Set aside and
heat the remainder of the olive oil in a large saucepan
over medium heat. Add the garlic and collard greens and
cook 5 – 10 minutes or until tender, stirring regularly.
Add the mustard and vinegar mixture and toss to coat
the greens. Transfer the greens to a serving bowl, top
with crumbled bacon and serve at once.

Tomato and Cheese Tart

Number of servings: 6

Ingredients:

The dough:
1 ½ cups all-purpose flour
6 tbsp unsalted butter, cold, cut into 1/2" pieces
2 tbsp olive oil (plus more as needed)
1 tbsp water
½ tsp salt
½ tsp pepper
The filling:
6 ounces Camembert cheese, cut into 1/8" thick slices
½ cup grated Gruyere or Swiss cheese
4 Roma tomatoes, sliced 1/2" thick
¼ cup fresh parsley, chopped (use flat leaf Italian parsley if possible)
¼ cup fresh basil, chopped
2 cloves of garlic, minced
½ cup olive oil (use extra virgin olive oil)
1 tbsp Dijon mustard
1 tsp fresh rosemary, minced
2 tsp fresh thyme leaves
1 bay leaf, crumbled into very small pieces

Preparation:

Start by making the dough for your tart. Combine the flour, butter, salt and pepper using a pastry cutter or two knives until you create a coarse, mealy mixture. Mix in 2 tbsp olive oil and the water using a fork, mixing just until the mixture starts to hold together at the bottom – add another tbsp of olive oil if needed. Gather the dough into a ball and flatten it out into a disk; wrap it in plastic wrap and place in the refrigerator for 30 minutes to chill.

Next, preheat your oven to 375 F while you roll out the dough into a 14" circle. Place the dough in a tart pan (or 9" circular pie tin) and set aside. Spread the mustard on the bottom of the shell, followed by the shredded Gruyere or Swiss cheese. Next, place alternating layers of tomato and sliced Camembert over the Gruyere.

Mix together the rest of the olive oil, the herbs and the garlic in a small bowl. Brush about three fourths of the mixture on the tart. Bake the tart for 35 minutes, then remove from the oven, brush with the rest of the oil mixture and serve warm.

Spicy Corn and Sweet Potato Soup

Number of servings: 6

Ingredients:

2 ½ lbs. sweet potatoes, diced into 1" pieces
1 cup corn kernels, either fresh cut or frozen
4 cups vegetable broth
2 cups water
1 cup dry sherry
1 cup whole milk
2 jalapenos, diced (you may also seed them if you prefer a milder flavor)
1 large yellow onion, diced
4 cloves of garlic, minced
2 tbsp butter
1 tbsp olive oil
2 tsp chili powder
1 tsp poultry seasoning
salt and black pepper, to taste
thinly sliced green onions, for garnish

Preparation:

Heat the olive oil in a large, heavy saucepan or stock pot. Once the oil is hot, add the garlic and cook until aromatic, about one minute. Add the onion and jalapenos and cook for another 5 minutes or until the onions are tender, stirring occasionally.

Add the sweet potatoes and water. Bring the pot to a slow boil and continue simmering for about 15 minutes or until the sweet potatoes become tender. Puree the soup using a blender or food processor and return to the pot. Add the corn and vegetable broth and bring the soup back up to a slow boil for about 10 minutes. Add the butter, milk and sherry and reduce the heat to a simmer. Mix thoroughly to incorporate the milk, butter and sherry and keep on a low simmer until ready to serve.

Easy Caramelized Onion Pizza

Number of servings: 6

Ingredients:

1 large flat loaf of focaccia bread
2 medium yellow or red onions, thinly sliced
12 ounces crimini mushrooms, stems removed and sliced
6 Kalamata olives, pitted and halved
2 ounces dry white wine
6 tbsp ricotta cheese
5 tbsp olive oil
crushed red pepper, to taste

Preparation:

Start by preheating your oven to 350 F. Heat 2 tbsp of the olive oil in a large skillet for about 1 minute. Add the sliced onions and cook over medium heat until the onions start to caramelize – this will take roughly 20 minutes. Stir the onions occasionally to prevent them from burning. Add the wine about halfway through; this will keep them from drying out as well as adding flavor. Once the onions are caramelized, remove them from the pan and set aside.

Heat 2 tbsp olive oil for about 1 minute in a skillet (you can simply wipe out the skillet you caramelized the onions in and reuse it to cut down on clean up time afterwards). Add the mushrooms and cook for about 10 minutes, or until the mushrooms have released most of their water and are slightly browned.

Brush the focaccia with the remaining tbsp of olive oil. Spread the ricotta cheese over the focaccia and then layer the caramelized onions and sautéed mushrooms on top, followed by the olives. Bake the pizza for about 10 minutes; if you'd like the crust to be crisper, increase the heat to broil for another 2 – 3 minutes before removing from the oven and serving hot.

Roasted Squash & Kale Salad

Number of servings: 4 as a main course, 6 as a side dish

Ingredients:

1 medium-sized butternut squash
1 large bunch of lacinato kale (aka Tuscan kale or
dinosaur kale)
1 large shallot, minced
1 tbsp olive oil (use extra virgin olive oil)
Parmesan or Romano cheese
salt and black pepper, to taste
For the dressing:
1/3 cup olive oil (extra virgin)
3 tbsp balsamic vinegar or red wine vinegar
1 small shallot, minced

Preparation:

Start by preheating your oven to 350 F. Peel the squash,
cut in half and remove the seeds and pulp from the
middle cavity. Slice the squash into wedges about ½"
wide and arrange in a baking pan topped with minced
shallots. Drizzle the olive oil over the squash and season
with a little salt and black pepper. Bake the squash for
about 35 – 40 minutes, or until the edges are lightly

browned and the flesh has become tender.

While you roast the squash you can prepare the kale and the dressing. Wash the kale, pat dry and slice it into wide strips (about 1" wide). In a small bowl, whisk together the olive oil, vinegar and minced shallow and massage the dressing into the kale in a large bowl, using your hands – this softens the kale as well as helping the leaves to absorb the flavor of the dressing.

Slice the Parmesan or Romano into thin slices (a cheese planer is a good tool for this) and set aside. Once the squash is done, toss it with the kale and cheese while it's still warm to allow the dressing to coat the squash.

Broiled Salmon with Green Beans

Number of servings: 4

Ingredients:

4 salmon filets, about 4 - 5 ounces each
1 lb. green beans (fresh, not canned or frozen)
2 tbsp fresh ginger, peeled and crushed
2 jalapenos, sliced (may be seeded for a milder flavor)
1 bunch of watercress or arugula, washed and patted
dry
black pepper, to taste
For the salmon dressing:
2/3 cup toasted sesame oil
juice of 1 orange
2 tbsp soy sauce
2 tbsp honey (may use less or more to taste)
For the green bean dressing:
2/3 cup olive oil (use extra virgin olive oil)
2 cloves of garlic, crushed
1 tbsp Dijon mustard
1 tbsp cognac vinegar or white wine vinegar (apple cider
vinegar is also OK)
a pinch each of salt and black pepper

Preparation:

Rinse the green beans to remove any dirt and trim off the ends. Steam the green beans in a steamer basket over about 1" of boiling water for about five minutes, or until they're crisp-tender.

You can make your dressing while the beans are steaming. Peel and crush the garlic with a garlic press and place in a small bowl. Add the mustard and vinegar and then whisk in the olive oil until thoroughly combined. Toss with the green beans once they're finished steaming and set aside.

Now it's time to prepare the salmon filets. Turn your oven to broil and mix together the ingredients for the salmon dressing. Place the filets in a baking pan and pour half of the dressing over them. Peel and crush the ginger and slice the jalapenos, removing the seeds if you'd like less heat. Top the salmon filets with the crushed ginger and pepper slices and broil for about 5 minutes (adjust the cooking time depending on the thickness of the filets – about 8 minutes per inch of thickness is a good rule of thumb, but it's always better to err on the side of caution).

Lay a bed of watercress or arugula on a serving platter and place the cooked salmon filets on top. Spoon the remaining dressing over the filets and serve along with the green beans.

Kale and White Bean Stew

Number of servings: 4

Ingredients:

1 large bunch of kale (about 5 cups packed), washed and thinly sliced
1 lb. cannellini beans, cooked and drained (other small white beans may be substituted if needed)
1 lb. Roma tomatoes, diced
2 cups chicken or vegetable broth
4 cloves of garlic, minced
4 tbsp olive oil
1 tbsp apple cider vinegar
1 tsp each dried basil and dried thyme (or more, to taste)
½ tsp crushed red pepper
salt and black pepper, to taste
extra virgin olive oil and grated Romano or Parmesan cheese, for garnish

Preparation:

Heat the olive oil, minced garlic and crushed red pepper over medium heat in a stock pot or large, heavy saucepan for about 1 minute. Add the vinegar, chicken or vegetable broth and kale and bring to a boil. Reduce the heat to a simmer and add the thyme and basil. Cover and cook for about 5 minutes, or until the kale wilts. Add the tomatoes and beans and continue simmering, covered for 20 minutes. Taste and season with salt and black pepper. Serve hot in soup bowls with a drizzle of olive oil and a pinch of grated Romano or Parmesan cheese.

Baked Beets

Number of servings: 6

Ingredients:

4 medium-sized beets, sliced ¼ inch thick (peeling is optional)
½ cup water
¼ cup dry white wine (Sauvignon Blanc is a good choice for this recipe)
1 cup milk
3 tbsp butter
3 tbsp all-purpose flour
1 shallot, minced
salt and black pepper, to taste
a pinch of nutmeg

Preparation:

Start by preheating your oven to 425 F. Arrange the sliced beets in a large (9" x 13") baking dish and add the water. Cover the dish tightly with foil and bake for about 45 minutes or until the beets are tender.

After the beets have been in the oven for about half an hour, you can start to make a béchamel sauce. Melt the butter over medium heat in a saucepan and add the minced shallot once the butter has melted completely. Saute for 2 – 3 minutes or until softened. Add the flour and stir to form a roux. Whisk in the milk and then the wine slowly, adding just a little at a time. Once the milk and wine have been incorporated, bring the mixture to a slow boil – the sauce will start to thicken. Remove the sauce from heat and season to taste with salt and pepper and add a dash of nutmeg (or more, if desired).

Pour the sauce over the beets and continue to bake uncovered in the sauce for another 10 minutes or until the sauce bubbles and starts to turn golden brown around the edges. Remove from the oven, allow them to stand for a minute and then serve the beets while they're still hot.

Bean and Barley Vegetable Soup

Number of servings: 6

Ingredients:

1 small yellow or white onion, diced
2 celery stalks, diced
4 cloves garlic, minced
2 medium sized carrots, diced
1 cup uncooked barley
8 cups vegetable broth, beef broth or water
1 cup cooked white beans or pinto beans
½ cup crushed tomatoes (or tomato paste, if you don't
have fresh tomatoes on hand)
2 tbsp olive oil
1 tsp basil
1 tsp oregano
½ tsp thyme
2 bay leaves
salt and black pepper, to taste

Preparation:

Heat the olive oil in a stock pot and sauté the onions,
carrots, garlic and celery for 5 minutes, stirring
occasionally. Add the water or broth, along with all of

the other ingredients and bring the soup to a slow boil before reducing to a simmer. Simmer uncovered for 1 – 2 hours, stirring occasionally until the barley is tender. Season to taste with salt and black pepper before serving.

This recipe is very adaptable; if you'd like, you can add virtually any vegetables or cooked meat to the pot along with the broth. Feel free to experiment as long as you leave in the superfoods in this recipe – the tomatoes, onion and beans – to make sure it provides the maximum nutritional value.

Chickpeas and Mustard Greens with a Balsamic Glaze

Number of servings: 4 as a side dish, 2 as an entrée

Ingredients:

3 tightly packed cups of mustard greens, washed, patted dry and sliced
1 cup cooked chickpeas, drained and rinsed
1 small red onion, sliced thinly
4 cloves of garlic, sliced thinly
4 tbsp vegetable broth
2 tbsp balsamic vinegar
1 tsp soy sauce
½ tsp sugar
crushed red pepper, to taste

Preparation:

Cook the onion in a large, heavy saucepan with 1 tbsp of the vegetable broth over medium heat until it starts to soften and turn pink, about 4 minutes. Add the garlic, a little crushed red pepper and 1 more tbsp of broth and cook for one more minute, stirring regularly. Add the other 2 tbsp of broth and the mustard greens and continue to cook for 3 – 5 minutes, stirring regularly, until the greens are wilted. Remove the greens and onions with a slotted spoon and transfer to a serving plate, but leave any remaining cooking liquid in the saucepan.

Add the vinegar, soy sauce and sugar to the pan; if there's no broth left in the pan, add 2 more tbsp of broth. Add the chickpeas and cook over medium heat until the chickpeas are warmed through and the liquid is reduced by half. Remove the chickpeas from the pan with a slotted spoon and place on top of the greens and then pour the balsamic glaze over the greens and chickpeas. Serve hot with balsamic vinegar on the side.

Rigatoni with Walnuts, Italian Sausage and Broccoli Rabe

Number of servings: 4

Ingredients:

1 lb. rigatoni or penne pasta, preferably whole grain
4 Italian sausages (sweet or hot), with the casings removed
1 bunch broccoli rabe (rapini), trimmed and chopped coarsely
2 cups basil leaves, packed loosely
¾ cup olive oil (use extra virgin olive oil)
½ cup walnuts
½ cup ricotta cheese
4 cloves of garlic, peeled and trimmed
½ tsp salt
salt and black pepper, to taste

Preparation:

Start by preheating your oven to 300 F. Spread out the walnuts on a baking sheet and toast until they're slightly browned, about 7 minutes. Remove the toasted walnuts from the oven and allow them to cool completely before using.

Once the walnuts have cooled to room temperature, measure out ¼ cup of walnuts and place in a food processor. Add the basil leaves, garlic cloves and ¼ tsp salt. Process the ingredients, adding ½ cup of extra virgin olive oil to the mixture as it processes. Mix until the ingredients reach the right consistency for pesto (smooth, but not a puree).

Chop the rest of the toasted walnuts finely and set aside. In a large saucepan or stockpot, bring lightly salted water to a boil and add a splash of olive oil (this is to prevent the pot from boiling over as well as keeping the pasta from sticking together during cooking). Add the rigatoni and cook until it's slightly more tender than al dente. Drain the pasta and set aside.

While the water is boiling, heat 2 tbsp of olive oil in a large skillet. Once the olive oil is hot, add the Italian sausage to the skillet and cook, stirring regularly to break up the meat. Saute until the sausage is browned, about 5 minutes. Remove the sausage from the skillet and place in a small bowl, leaving the fat behind in the skillet.

Add the rest of the olive oil to the skillet and the broccoli rabe. Saute, stirring regularly, until the broccoli rabe is crisp-tender, about 3 minutes. Add a little water, reduce the heat to a simmer and cook, covered, for another 5 minutes until tender. Add ¼ tsp salt and a little black pepper, stir and return the Italian sausage to the pan; cook for another 1 – 2 minutes, until the sausage is heated through.

Toss the cooked rigatoni with the walnut pesto and season to taste with salt and black pepper. Divide the pasta among four individual plates and top with the broccoli rabe and sausage mixture, a little ricotta cheese and a sprinkling of chopped walnuts. Serve immediately.

Cabbage Rolls

Number of servings: 6

Ingredients:

6 large red cabbage leaves
1 cup chopped mixed mushrooms – straw mushrooms, enoki mushrooms, crimini, etc.
1 cup bean sprouts, rinsed and patted dry
½ of a small carrot, slivered
½ tsp rice vinegar
a pinch of salt
a little bit of sesame oil, for sautéing
For the sauce:
2 ½ tbsp water or vegetable broth
½ tbsp hoisin sauce
a dash of toasted sesame oil
a pinch of sugar
black pepper and crushed red pepper, to taste

Preparation:

Blanch the cabbage leaves in boiling water for 2 minutes, then place in cold water. Drain well, pat dry and set aside. Mix together the mushrooms, sprouts, carrot, rice vinegar and salt in a medium sized bowl.

Heat a little sesame oil in a skillet or wok; once it's hot, add the mushroom mix and cook for 2 – 3 minutes, stirring regularly. Divide the filling among the 6 blanched cabbage leaves and roll up tightly to seal.

Place the cabbage rolls in a steamer basket over about 1" of boiling water and steam, covered for about 5 minutes. While the cabbage rolls are steaming, whisk together the ingredients for the sauce. Remove the cabbage rolls from the steamer and serve, hot, topped with the sauce.

Steak with Roast Vegetables

Number of servings: 4

Ingredients:

4 small sirloin steaks, 4 – 6 ounces each
4 small beets, sliced into wedges
4 small sweet potatoes, cut into 1" chunks
1 medium yellow or white onion, peeled and quartered
1 bulb of garlic, peeled and cloves separated
4 tbsp olive oil (use extra virgin olive oil)
2 tbsp balsamic vinegar or red wine vinegar
A few sprigs of rosemary
1 tightly packed cup of baby spinach leaves
1 tbsp ground horseradish
2 tbsp lemon juice
salt and black pepper, to taste

Preparation:

Preheat your oven to 400 F. Place the vegetables except
for the garlic in a large baking dish and drizzle with half
of the olive oil and the balsamic or red wine vinegar.
Bake for 15 minutes and then add the garlic cloves and
rosemary. Bake for another 30 minutes or until the
vegetables are tender and beginning to caramelize.

Transfer the roasted vegetables to a large bowl and stir together with the baby spinach leaves.

Season the steaks with salt and black pepper and sear in a hot skillet with a little oil, cooking about 2 minutes per side; set aside to rest for 5 minutes. Mix the other 2 tbsp of olive oil with the horseradish and the lemon juice, along with a pinch each of salt and black pepper.

Divide the roasted vegetables among four individual plates and place the steaks on top. Drizzle the sauce over each plate and serve at once.

Spicy Beef Soup

Number of servings: 6 - 8

Ingredients:

1lb lean ground beef
4 cups chopped kale
4 cups shredded Savoy cabbage
3 large tomatoes, diced
6 cloves of garlic, minced or crushed
2 jalapeno peppers, diced (remove seeds for a milder taste)
1 medium sized yellow onion, diced
1 large red bell pepper, sliced
1 cup sliced mushrooms (crimini or button)
1 cup sliced okra (optional)
4 cups water
juice of 1 lemon
3 tbsp apple cider vinegar
3 tbsp soy sauce or Bragg's liquid aminos
2 tbsp olive oil (use extra virgin olive oil)
2 tsp thyme
Salt and black pepper, to taste

Preparation:

In a large, heavy stock pot, sauté the onions, garlic, jalapeno peppers and okra in 2 tbsp olive oil until the onions and garlic are fragrant and begin to turn translucent, about 3 minutes over medium heat. Stir regularly to prevent burning.

Add the ground beef, lemon juice and soy sauce and continue cooking until the ground beef is cooked through, 5 – 7 minutes. Add the diced tomatoes and water and bring to a low boil. Add the Savoy cabbage, kale and mushrooms and reduce to a simmer. Cook, covered, for 30 – 45 minutes; keep warm until ready to serve.

Slow Cooker Beef and Sweet Potato Curry

Number of servings: 6

Ingredients:

1 ½ lbs. top sirloin, diced
1 large sweet potato, cut into roughly 1" cubes
2 cups cauliflower florets
1 cup green beans, rinsed, trimmed and cut into halves crosswise
1 large yellow onion, diced
1 ½ cups beef stock
2/3 cup coconut milk
3 tbsp red curry paste (green curry paste may be substituted, if you prefer)
2 tbsp peanut butter
1 tsp cumin
1 tsp cinnamon
3 cups cooked brown rice, for serving

Preparation:

This recipe is incredibly easy to make. Simply prepare all of the ingredients with the exceptions of the cauliflower florets and green beans and place them in a slow cooker or crock pot and cook on low, covered, for 7 hours.

After the curry has been cooking for almost 7 hours, prepare your cauliflower and green beans, add to the pot and cook for another hour – which gives you plenty of time to cook the brown rice. Serve hot over brown rice.

Side Dishes and Appetizers

Roasted Eggplant Salad

Number of servings: varies

Ingredients:

The eggplant:
3 large eggplants
2 roasted red peppers, diced
2 green bell peppers, cored, seeded and diced small
4 cloves of garlic, minced
2 Roma tomatoes, diced
½ cup parsley (use flat leaved Italian parsley), chopped
2 tbsp fresh basil, chopped
1 tbsp olive oil (use extra virgin olive oil for this recipe)
juice of 3 lemons
salt and black pepper, to taste
crushed red pepper, to taste (optional)
The yogurt sauce:
2 cups plain Greek yogurt
½ cup peeled, diced cucumber
1 tbsp fresh mint, chopped
2 tsp olive oil
juice of 1 lemon

a pinch of salt

Preparation:

Start by heating your oven to 450 F and lining a baking sheet with foil. Pierce the eggplants with a knife or fork in a few spots. Place the eggplants on the foil lined baking sheet and bake for 35 – 40 minutes or until they collapse. Remove the roasted eggplants from the oven and allow them to cool until they're safe to handle.

Cut the eggplants in half lengthwise. Scoop out the flesh (a grapefruit spoon may be helpful for this task) and transfer into a bowl. Discard the skins. Add the juice of 2 lemons to the bowl and allow the eggplant to marinate in the juice for 10 minutes.

Transfer the eggplant into a fine strainer and using the back of a large spoon, press the eggplant against the mesh to force out as much moisture as possible. Remove the eggplant from the strainer and chop coarsely. Transfer the eggplant back to the bowl and add the diced peppers, tomatoes, minced garlic, chopped parsley, basil, extra virgin olive oil and the juice of another lemon. Set the mixture aside.

Now you can make your yogurt sauce; this part is a lot

easier than preparing the eggplant. Simply place all of the ingredients in a bowl and mix well to combine. Serve the eggplant salad along with the yogurt sauce and whole wheat pita bread or pita chips.

Pomegranate Carrots

Number of servings: 4

Ingredients

3 ½ cups of carrots, sliced into ¼" thick rounds

1 tbsp olive oil

1 tsp coriander

1 tsp salt

1 cup pomegranate juice, unsweetened

a pinch of cinnamon

black pepper, to taste

chopped fresh parsley, for garnish (use flat leaved Italian parsley if possible)

Preparation:

Heat the olive oil in a large skillet or medium saucepan over medium high heat. Once the oil is hot, add the sliced carrots to the pan. Cook for 5 minutes, stirring regularly. Add the salt and coriander, stir and continue cooking for another 1 - 2 minutes, stirring occasionally. Add the cinnamon and pomegranate juice and reduce the heat to medium. Simmer, uncovered, over medium-low heat for 15 – 20 minutes, stirring regularly until the juice has reduced to a glaze and the carrots are tender. Serve hot topped with chopped parsley.

Broccoli with Bell Peppers

Number of servings: 6

Ingredients:

4 cups broccoli florets (fresh, not frozen); you can also
include sliced broccoli stems in the dish if you like
1 medium sized yellow bell pepper, thinly sliced
1 medium sized red bell pepper, thinly sliced
1 medium sized tomato, diced
4 cloves of garlic, minced
1 tbsp olive oil (use extra virgin olive oil)
1 tsp oregano
6 cups water
1 tbsp grated Parmesan or Romano cheese
salt and black pepper, to taste

Preparation:

Bring 6 cups of water to boil in a large saucepan. Add the
broccoli florets to the pan and boil, covered for 2
minutes. Drain and transfer the broccoli to a bowl of
cold water immediately; allow the broccoli to cool in the
water for a minute, then drain and pat dry with a clean
kitchen towel.

Heat the olive oil in a large skillet. Once the oil is hot, sauté the peppers until crisp-tender, about 3 minutes, stirring occasionally. Add the blanched broccoli florets, minced garlic and oregano and cook for another 2 minutes, until the garlic becomes fragrant and the broccoli is almost heated through. Add the diced tomatoes and heat through, another 2 minutes. Season to taste with salt and black pepper and divide among individual plates, sprinkle with a little Parmesan or Romano cheese and serve hot.

Leeks with Vinaigrette

Number of servings: 6

Ingredients:

6 leeks (discard the dark green tops)
3 cloves of garlic, sliced thinly
6 – 8 sprigs of fresh thyme
juice of 3 lemons
4 tbsp olive oil (use extra virgin olive oil)
1 ½ tbsp salt
2 tsp Dijon mustard
salt and black pepper, to taste
extra sprigs of thyme, for garnish

Preparation:

Slice off the dark green tops and the very bottoms of the leeks, halve lengthwise and place in a large bowl of cold water. Allow the leeks to soak at least half an hour to remove dirt and grit – rinse the leeks thoroughly between soaking and using.

While the leeks soak, bring 4 quarts of water, the sliced garlic, 1 ½ tbsp salt and the juice of 2 lemons to a boil in a large stockpot. Reduce the heat and simmer until the leeks are soaked and rinsed. Add the leeks to the pot and continue simmering for 15 – 20 minutes or until the leeks are tender. Drain the cooking liquid and pat the leeks dry with a clean kitchen towel.

In a small bowl, whisk together the Dijon mustard, the juice of 1 lemon and olive oil, along with a pinch of salt and black pepper. Toss the leeks with the lemon dressing to coat and serve, topped with a little freshly ground black pepper and thyme sprigs.

Chickpea and Sweet Potato Dip

Number of servings: 6+ (this recipe makes about 2 ½ cups of dip)

Ingredients:

1 can (15 or 16 ounces) of chickpeas, drained and rinsed (or the equivalent amount of homemade cooked chickpeas)
1 medium sized sweet potato, well scrubbed
3 cloves of garlic, crushed
½ cup olive oil (use extra virgin olive oil), plus 1 tbsp for drizzling
salt and black pepper, to taste
hot sauce, to taste

Preparation:

Pierce the sweet potato in several places with a fork or knife and bake at 425 F for about 45 minutes or until tender when poked with a fork. Remove from heat, slice in half lengthwise (this will help it cool faster) and allow it to cool until it's safe to handle.

Once the sweet potato is cool enough to touch, drain and rinse the chickpeas and add to a food processor along with the crushed garlic and a little salt. Scoop the flesh from the sweet potato and add to the chickpeas, garlic and salt. Process on low speed, adding olive oil (and hot sauce, if using) to the mixture little by little until the dip has become a smooth puree.

Transfer the dip to a serving bowl and drizzle with 1 tbsp of olive oil. Serve at room temperature.

Quinoa Salad with Kale and Avocado

Number of servings: 4 – 6

Ingredients:

2/3 cup dry quinoa
1 1/3 cups water
1 large bunch of lacinato kale (aka Tuscan or dinosaur kale), torn into manageable bite-sized pieces
1 avocado, diced
1 small cucumber, diced
1 small red bell pepper, diced
¼ cup diced red onion
2 tbsp feta cheese, crumbled (or more to taste)
For the dressing:
¼ cup olive oil (use extra virgin olive oil)
Juice of 1- 2 lemons (about 2 tbsp)
2 tbsp Dijon mustard
1 tsp salt
black pepper, to taste

Preparation:

Add the quinoa and water to a saucepan and bring to a boil and then reduce to a simmer and cook, covered, for about 15 minutes or until the water has been absorbed and the quinoa is tender. Remove from heat, uncover and allow the quinoa to cool.

Steam the kale in a steamer basket over a little (about 1") of boiling water in a large saucepan, covered. Steam for about 2 minutes, just until wilted and remove from heat. Transfer the kale to a large bowl and allow it to cool to room temperature before topping with the quinoa, avocado slices, diced red bell pepper, onion, cucumber and crumbled feta cheese.

In a small bowl, whisk together the mustard, olive oil, lemon juice, salt and black pepper until thoroughly combined. Pour the dressing over the salad and serve.

Pumpkin and Flax Seed Dip

Number of servings: varies

Ingredients:

1 cup pumpkin seeds, roasted and lightly salted
1/3 cup flax seeds
1 small jalapeno or Serrano pepper
1 small shallot
2 cloves of garlic

2 tbsp chopped cilantro

1 tsp cumin

½ tsp ground coriander

juice and zest of 1 orange

juice and zest of 2 lemons

2 tbsp mayonnaise

black pepper, to taste

olive oil and paprika, for garnish

Preparation:

Add the garlic, shallot and jalapeno or Serrano pepper to a food processor and mince. Add the pumpkin and flax seeds and process again, before adding the chopped cilantro, mayonnaise, citrus juice and zest and spices and blending until the mixture becomes a smooth puree; add a little olive oil if needed. Transfer the dip to a bowl, drizzle with olive oil and sprinkle with paprika before serving.

Spinach Salad with Fruit and Almonds

Number of servings: 4 – 6

Ingredients:

1 (6 ounce) bag of baby spinach
1 cup strawberries, trimmed and sliced into quarters
1 cup fresh raspberries or blueberries
1 cup fresh pineapple chunks
½ cup sliced almonds
½ cup dressing, your choice (a lemon vinaigrette is a good choice)

Preparation:
 Combine all ingredients in a large bowl and serve.

Roasted Brussels Sprouts

Number of servings: 4

Ingredients:

1 lb. Brussels sprouts, washed, trimmed and cut in half
1 tbsp olive oil
2 tsp honey
1 tsp salt
black pepper, to taste
crushed red pepper, to taste (optional)

Preparation:

Preheat your oven to 450 F. Lightly oil a large baking pan or sheet. In a large bowl, toss the Brussels sprouts with honey, olive oil, salt, black pepper and red pepper. Transfer to the baking pan or sheet, forming a single layer. Bake for about 25 minutes, or until browned and serve hot.

Roasted Garlic Soup

Number of servings: 4 - 6

Ingredients:

2 large heads of garlic, unpeeled
4 cloves of garlic, crushed
1 large potato, cubed
2 medium yellow onions, minced
2 medium sized carrots, minced
4 cups chicken or vegetable stock
½ cup dry white wine (preferably Chardonnay or Chenin Blanc)
¼ cup heavy cream
3 tbsp olive oil
1 tbsp butter
2 bay leaves
1 tsp white pepper (optional)
salt and black pepper, to taste

Preparation:

The first step is to roast the garlic. Preheat your oven to 350 F. Use a bread knife or other serrated knife to slice off the top of the garlic heads and expose the tip of each clove. Place the garlic on a piece of aluminum foil and drizzle with 2 tbsp olive oil. Add the bay leaves to the foil and fold it up, sealing the edges to form a packet. Bake the foil-wrapped garlic for 45 minutes. Remove the roasted garlic from the oven and allow it to cool until it's safe to handle. Squeeze the garlic heads into a small bowl and discard the bay leaves and garlic husks.

Now you're ready to start making your broth. Heat the butter and the rest of the olive oil in a large, heavy saucepan or stock pot over medium heat. Add the onions and cook until they turn translucent, stirring occasionally. Add the carrots and cook for another 5 minutes. Add the crushed garlic and cook until it becomes fragrant, about another 2 minutes.

Add the diced potato, stock, wine, roasted garlic and salt and pepper to taste. Bring the soup to a boil and then reduce the heat to medium-low and simmer, covered, for another 40 minutes.

Once the soup is cooked, puree it in batches using a blender or food processor until smooth. Return the pureed soup to the pan and whisk in the cream. Heat on medium heat until warmed through, but do not allow the soup to come to a boil – reduce heat to low and keep the soup warm until you're ready to serve.

Bagna Cauda

Number of servings: varies

Ingredients:

¾ cup olive oil (use extra virgin olive oil)
10 anchovy fillets, drained and rinsed well
6 cloves of garlic, peeled
6 tbsp butter
black pepper, to taste

Preparation:

Place the anchovy fillets, butter and garlic in a food processor and process until blended (this should take about 1 minute). While the processor is still running, add the oil a little at a time until it's thoroughly mixed in.

Transfer the mixture to a small saucepan over medium-low heat and cook just until it's heated through. Remove from heat, transfer to a bowl and serve hot with raw vegetables and/or crackers.

Red Bean Dip

Number of servings: varies

Ingredients:

1 can (15 – 16 ounces) small red beans or kidney beans, drained and rinsed
½ cup sliced avocado (about ½ an avocado)
½ cup Greek yogurt
1 tbsp olive oil (use extra virgin olive oil), plus extra for garnish
1 tbsp sliced green onions (use just the green parts for this recipe)
1 tsp cumin
salt and black pepper, to taste

Preparation:

Place the red or kidney beans, Greek yogurt, olive oil, pepper, cumin and a little salt and pepper in a food processor. Blend the mixture until smooth. Transfer the dip to a serving bowl and garnish with a drizzle of olive oil and sliced green onions. Serve at room temperature or cold with crackers or tortilla chips.

Quinoa Salad with Lemon Vinaigrette

Number of servings: 4 - 6

Ingredients:

2 cups cooked quinoa, cooled to room temperature
1 small red onion, diced
1 avocado, sliced
1 small orange peeled, separated into segments and
chopped
1 cup cooked black beans, canned or homemade,
drained and rinsed
1 cup pomegranate arils (this is about the amount you'll
find in one pomegranate)
1/3 cup corn kernels, fresh cut or frozen and thawed
1/3 cup chopped cilantro
salt and black pepper, to taste
For the dressing:
Juice of 2 lemons
6 tbsp olive oil (use extra virgin olive oil)
2 cloves of garlic, minced
a pinch of sugar
salt and black pepper, to taste

Preparation:

Combine all of the ingredients for the dressing in a small jar and shake to mix.

Add the cooked quinoa, red onion, orange, avocado, beans, corn, pomegranate and cilantro to a bowl and stir to combine. Pour the dressing over the salad, stir again to mix well and season to taste with salt and black pepper. Stir and serve at room temperature or chill and serve cold.

Cranberry Salsa

Number of servings: varies

Ingredients:

2 (14 – 16 ounce) cans of cranberry sauce (only use the whole berry kind)
1 small white onion, diced
2 jalapeno peppers and 4 – 6 Serrano peppers (use more or less to taste)
juice of 3 limes
4 green onions, trimmed and sliced

Preparation:

Add the white onion, green onion, jalapeno peppers and Serrano peppers to a food processor and process until finely chopped. Transfer the chopped onions and peppers to a large bowl. Add the two cans of cranberry sauce and stir well to combine. Add the lime juice, stir again and chill for 1 – 2 hours or overnight to allow the flavors to combine before serving.

Breakfast

Blueberry-Walnut Muffins

Number of servings: 6 large or 12 regular size muffins

Ingredients:

1 ½ cups blueberries (fresh or frozen)
1 cup rolled oats
½ cup all-purpose flour
½ cup whole wheat flour
½ cup applesauce (unsweetened)
½ cup plain yogurt
½ cup chopped walnuts
2 egg whites (from large eggs)
1 large whole egg
2 tbsp maple syrup
1 tbsp baking powder
1 tsp baking soda
1 tsp vanilla extract
1 tsp cinnamon

Preparation:

Preheat your oven to 400 F and line your muffin tins with muffin papers.

In a large bowl, mix the yogurt, egg, egg whites, maple syrup and vanilla extract until thoroughly combined. In another large bowl, mix together the flours, oats, baking powder, baking soda, cinnamon and walnuts and blueberries.

Mix together the dry and wet ingredients and mix just until the dry ingredients are moistened. Divide the muffin batter among your muffin tins and bake for about 25 minutes, or until the tops are dry and golden brown. Turn the muffins out of the tins and cool on a wire rack before serving.

Oatmeal-Blueberry Pancakes

Number of servings: varies

Ingredients:

2 cups blueberries, fresh or frozen (thaw first if using frozen)
1 ½ cups rolled oats
1 cup all-purpose flour
½ cup whole wheat flour
1 ½ cups milk
1 cup buttermilk
¼ cup sugar
2 large eggs plus 2 egg whites from large eggs
1 tbsp lemon juice
1 tsp baking soda
1 tsp baking powder
1 tsp cinnamon
½ tsp salt
cooking spray

Preparation:

Mix together the buttermilk and oats in a bowl; allow the oats to hydrate in the buttermilk for about 15 minutes. In a separate, medium sized bowl, mix the all-purpose and whole wheat flour, the baking soda and baking powder, the sugar, salt and cinnamon. In another small bowl, whisk together the two eggs and the two egg whites, then mix in the milk. Pour the wet ingredients into the dry ingredients and stir to combine.

Heat a nonstick skillet coated with cooking spray over medium-high heat. Once the skillet is hot, you can start making pancakes. About half a cup of batter should be enough for one pancake. Cook each pancake for about 2 minutes per side. Transfer finished pancakes to a place and cover to keep warm until you make your way through the batter.

While the pancakes are cooking, you can make your blueberry topping. Add the blueberries, lemon juice and sugar to a saucepan and cook over medium heat until the berries start to fall apart, about 5 minutes. Add the cinnamon, stir and remove from heat. Serve the pancakes immediately topped with the blueberry sauce.

Apple – Flax Seed Muffins

Number of servings: 6

Ingredients:

1 ½ cups pastry flour (preferably whole wheat)
¾ cup water
½ cup applesauce
½ cup sugar
¼ cup flax seeds, plus a little extra for sprinkling on top
½ of a Granny Smith apple, peeled, sliced thin and chopped into small pieces
1 tsp baking powder
1 tsp salt
1 tsp cinnamon

Preparation:

Preheat your oven to 400 degrees. Grease or flour your muffin tin. In a medium sized bowl, mix the dry ingredients except for the sugar. Make a well in the center of the dry ingredients and add the chopped apple pieces, applesauce and sugar. Mix well to moisten the ingredients evenly. Distribute the batter evenly among 6 muffin tins, sprinkle with flax seeds and bake for 20 minutes, or until the tops are firm and golden brown.

Remove from the oven, turn the muffins out of the tins and allow to cool thoroughly before serving.

An Apple a Day Smoothie

An apple a day is easy to eat in this delicious apple smoothie with bananas and orange juice. Makes 2 servings.

What You'll Need:

1 apple (Gala, peeled, cored, chopped)
1 banana (frozen, peeled, chopped)
1/2 cup of orange juice
1/4 cup of ice
1/4 cup of milk

How to Make It:

Combine the 1 apple (Gala, peeled, cored, chopped), 1 banana (frozen, peeled, chopped), 1/2 cup of orange juice, 1/4 cup of ice, and 1/4 cup of milk in a blender or food processor and blend until smooth. Pour into 2 tall glasses.

Apple Bran Muffins with Streusel

Here is a delicious and delightful muffin for breakfast. Makes 1 dozen muffins.

What You'll Need:

2 apples (peeled, cored, chopped)

2 eggs

2 1/4 cups of flour (all purpose, divided)

1 cup of brown sugar (divided)

1 cup of milk

1 cup of wheat bran (unprocessed)

1/2 cup of canola oil

2 tablespoons of butter (cold, crumbled)

1 tablespoon of baking powder

1 1/2 teaspoons of cinnamon (ground, divided)

1 teaspoon of salt

1/2 teaspoon of baking soda

How to Make It:

Prep: Preheat the oven to 375 degrees Fahrenheit. Add cupcake liners to 12 muffin cups.

Combine the 2 cups of flour (all purpose), 1 cup of wheat bran (unprocessed), 3/4 cup of brown sugar, 1 tablespoon of baking powder, 1 teaspoons of cinnamon (ground, divided), 1 teaspoon of salt, and 1/2 teaspoon of baking soda. In a separate bowl add the eggs and beat with a whisk and combine with the 1 cup of milk and 1/2 cup of canola oil. Add the dry ingredients into the web ingredients. Fold in the 2 apples (peeled, cored, chopped) and mix. Divide the batter into the 12 cupcake paper lined muffin cups. Combine 1/4 cups of flour (all purpose, divided), 1/4 cup of brown sugar (divided), and the 2 tablespoons of butter (cold, crumbled) in a bowl. Divide it over the 12 muffins. Bake in hot oven for about 27 minutes, muffins are done when toothpick inserted in the middle comes out clean.

Apple Cinnamon Bread with Raisins

A slice of this bread tastes great for breakfast. Makes 1 loaf.

What You'll Need:

2 eggs
1 1/2 cups of apple (grated)
1 1/2 cups of flour (all-purpose)
1 cup of oats (rolled)
2/3 cup of brown sugar (packed)
1/4 cup of canola oil
1/4 cup of milk
1/4 cup of raisins
1/4 cup of walnuts (chopped)
2 teaspoons of baking powder
1 1/4 teaspoon of cinnamon (ground)
1 teaspoon of salt
1/4 teaspoon of baking soda
1/4 teaspoon of nutmeg (ground)

How to Make It:

Prep: Preheat the oven to 350 degrees Fahrenheit. Spray a loaf pan with cooking spray.

Combine the 1 1/2 cups of flour (all-purpose), 1 cup of oats (rolled), 2/3 cup of brown sugar (packed), 2 teaspoons of baking powder, 1 1/4 teaspoon of cinnamon (ground), 1 teaspoon of salt, 1/4 teaspoon of baking soda, and 1/4 teaspoon of nutmeg (ground) in a bowl. Beat the 2 eggs with a whisk and add to the dry ingredients along with 1 1/2 cups of apple (grated), 1/4 cup of canola oil, 1/4 cup of milk, 1/4 cup of raisins, and 1/4 cup of walnuts (chopped). Batter will be lumpy, do not over stir. Pour into the loaf pan and bake for about 57 minutes. Cool on a wire rack before removing from pan.

Apple Cinnamon Toast

This is a delicious and quick breakfast. Makes 2 servings.

What You'll Need:

2 slices of whole grain bread
1 apple (peeled, cored, chopped)
2 teaspoons of brown sugar (light)
Apple Syrup (recipe below)
Cinnamon (ground)

Apple Syrup:
1 1/4 cups of apple juice (all natural)
1 tablespoon of cornstarch
1/4 teaspoon of nutmeg (ground)
1/4 teaspoon + more of cinnamon (ground)

How to Make It:

To make the apple syrup: Combine the 1 1/4 cups of apple juice (all natural), 1 tablespoon of cornstarch, 1/4 teaspoon of nutmeg (ground), and 1/4 teaspoon + more of cinnamon (ground) in a saucepan over high heat. Stir with a whisk and bring to a boil. Turn to low and cook for 5 minutes. Store in a closed contain in the refrigerator. Good on pancakes and in this recipe.

To make the toast:

Add the 1 apple (peeled, cored, chopped) and a tablespoon of the apple syrup in a double boiler and boil water for 10 minutes or until apples are tender. Toast the 2 slices of whole grain bread. Add the "cooked" apples on top of each slice, drizzle with apple syrup and sprinkle with ground cinnamon.

Baked Cranberry Oatmeal

This is the classic oatmeal with a few twists including cranberries and fresh from the oven. Makes 8 servings.

What You'll Need:

2 eggs
3 cups of oats (rolled)
1 cup of brown sugar
1 cup of milk
3/4 cup of cranberries (dried)
1/2 cup of butter (melted)
2 teaspoons of baking powder
2 teaspoons of cinnamon (ground)
2 teaspoons of vanilla extract
1 teaspoon of salt

How to Make It:

Prep: Preheat the oven to 350 degrees Fahrenheit.

Combine the 3 cups of oats (rolled), 1 cup of brown sugar, 2 teaspoons of baking powder, 2 teaspoons of cinnamon (ground), and 1 teaspoon of salt. Beat the 2 eggs in a cup with a whisk and add to the mixture along with the 1 cup of milk, 1/2 cup of butter (melted), and 2 teaspoons of vanilla extract. Fold in the 3/4 cup of cranberries (dried). Pour the mixture into a 9x13 inch baking dish and bake in the hot oven for 40 minutes. Let cool for a couple of minutes before serving.

Blackberry Smoothie

This delicious meal in a drink contains not only blackberries but also strawberries, bananas and orange juice. Makes 4 servings.

What You'll Need:

12 blackberries (fresh)
1 banana
2 cups of ice
1 cup of blackberries
1/2 cup of strawberries
1/3 cup of orange juice
1 teaspoon of honey

How to Make It:

Combine 1 banana, 2 cups of ice, 1 cup of blackberries, 1/2 cup of strawberries, 1/3 cup of orange juice, and 1 teaspoon of honey in a blender or food process and blend until smooth. Pour into 4 tall glasses and garnish with 3 fresh blackberries.

Blueberry Apple Pancakes

These are so good you will not miss the fact they are not made from processed flours. Makes 7 pancakes.

What You'll Need:

3 1/2 cups of vanilla rice milk
2 cups of blueberries
2 cups of oat flour
2 cups of spelt four
1/4 cup of applesauce
1/4 cup of flaxseed meal (ground)
2 tablespoons of agave nectar
2 tablespoons of baking powder
1 1/2 tablespoons of vanilla extract
1/2 teaspoon of salt

How to Make It:

Combine the 2 cups of oat flour, 2 cups of spelt four, 1/4 cup of flaxseed meal (ground), 2 tablespoons of baking powder, and 1/2 teaspoon of salt in a bowl. In a separate bowl, combine the 3 1/2 cups of vanilla rice milk, 1/4 cup of applesauce, 2 tablespoons of agave nectar, and 1 1/2 tablespoons of vanilla extract. Gradually add the wet ingredients into the dry. Stir until barely combined, set aside for about 15 minutes. Meanwhile spray the griddle or a skillet with cooking spray and turn heat to medium. Ladle the batter onto the hot surface and sprinkle several blueberries over the top as the pancake cooks. Flip after 3 minutes and cook for another 3 minutes. Repeat until all the batter is gone.

Cherry Oatmeal Bars

Sweet enough to be a dessert and nutritious enough to be for breakfast. Makes 24 bars.

What You'll Need:

1.5 cans of sweetened condensed milk (14 oz. per can)
2 cups of almonds (sliced)
2 cups of apricots (dried, chopped)
2 cups of cherries (dried)
2 cups of coconut (flakes, sweetened)
1 cup of flour (all purpose)
1 cup of oats (old fashioned)
3/4 cup of brown sugar (packed, light)
1/2 cup of butter
1/4 teaspoon of salt

How to Make It:

Preheat oven to 325 degrees Fahrenheit. Place rack to lowest position. Spray a 9x13 inch baking pan with cooking spray.

Combine the 1 cup of flour (all purpose), 1 cup of oats (old fashioned), 3/4 cup of brown sugar (packed, light), and 1/4 teaspoon of salt in a bowl. Take 1 1/2 cups of this oat mixture and pat into the bottom of the 9x13 pan. In a separate bowl combine the 2 cups of almonds (sliced), 2 cups of apricots (dried, chopped), 2 cups of cherries (dried), 2 cups of coconut (flakes, sweetened), and 1.5 cans of sweetened condensed milk (14 oz. per can). Spread the fruit mixture over the crust in the pan. Sprinkle the remaining oat mixture over the top and gently press down to form a top crust using a spatula. Bake in the hot oven for half an hour. Cool completely before cutting into 24 bars.

Energy Nut Bars

Enjoy a nice "bar" for breakfast, feels like candy but is packed with nutrition. Makes 30 bars.

What You'll Need:

4 egg whites
2 cups of milk (nonfat dry powder)
2 cups of rice cereal (crispy brown)
1 1/2 cups of oats (rolled)
1 cup of almonds (blanched)
1 cup of honey
1 cup of walnuts
3/4 cup of canola oil
1/2 cup of chocolate chips (semisweet, miniature)
1/2 cup of raisins
1/2 cup of soy nuts
1/2 cup of wheat germ
1/3 cup of flax seed meal
1 tablespoon of cinnamon (ground)
2 teaspoons of vanilla extract
1/2 teaspoon of salt

How to Make It:

Prep: Preheat the oven to 325 degrees Fahrenheit. Add

a sheet of foil to a baking sheet and spray it lightly with cooking spray.

Combine the 1 1/2 cups of oats (rolled), 1 cup of almonds (blanched), 1 cup of walnuts, and 1/2 cup of soy nuts in a blender or food processor and finely grind. Add to a large mixing bowl and combine with the 2 cups of milk (nonfat dry powder), 2 cups of rice cereal (crispy brown), 1/2 cup of chocolate chips (semisweet, miniature), 1/2 cup of raisins, 1/2 cup of wheat germ, 1/3 cup of flax seed meal, 1 tablespoon of cinnamon (ground), and 1/2 teaspoon of salt with a whisk. In a separate small bowl, beat the 4 egg whites until froth forms and combine with the 3/4 cup of canola oil and 2 teaspoons of vanilla extract. Add to the dry ingredients, mixing well. Press into the foil lined baking sheet and bake in the hot oven for 20 minutes. Let pan cool for 10 minutes, and then loosen the bars by lifting out of the pan by the foil, carefully. Cut into 30 bars. Cool completely before serving. Store in a sealed plastic bag or airtight container.

Granola Bars

A deliciously sweet and crunchy granola bar makes a perfect and filling breakfast. Makes 12 bars.

What You'll Need:

3 cups of oats (rolled)
3/4 cup of honey
3/4 cup of peanut butter (chunky)
1/2 cup of chocolate chips (semi-sweet)
1/2 cup of walnuts
1/3 cup of apricots (dried)
1/3 cup of prunes
1/3 cup of raisins
1/4 cup of sunflower seeds
2 tablespoons of wheat germ
1 tablespoon of sesame seeds
1/2 teaspoon of vanilla extract
1/8 teaspoon of salt

How to Make It:

Prep: Preheat the oven to 350 degrees Fahrenheit. Spray a 9x13 inch baking pan with cooking spray.

Combine the 3 cups of oats (rolled), 1/4 cup of

sunflower seeds, 2 tablespoons of wheat germ, 1 tablespoon of sesame seeds, and 1/8 teaspoon of salt together and set the bowl aside. Combine the 3/4 cup of honey, 3/4 cup of peanut butter (chunky), and 1/2 teaspoon of vanilla extract in a smaller bowl. Carefully add the honey mixture into the oat mixture the dough will be thick. Fold in the 1/2 cup of chocolate chips (semi-sweet), 1/2 cup of walnuts, 1/3 cup of apricots (dried), 1/3 cup of prunes, and 1/3 cup of raisins. Try to combine evenly. Spread the dough into the prepared 9x13 baking pan, press with fingers to make the top even. Bake in the hot oven for 20 minutes, or until the top turns a golden brown. Cool on a wire rack before cutting into 12 bars.

Apple Honey Muffins

This delicious treat makes an awesome breakfast. Makes a dozen muffins.

What You'll Need:

2 egg whites
2 cups of whole wheat flour
1 cup of apples (chopped)
3/4 cup of milk
1/4 cup of canola oil
1/4 cup of honey

1 tablespoon of baking powder

1 teaspoon of cinnamon (ground)

1/2 teaspoon of salt

How to Make It:

Prep: Preheat the oven to 375 degrees Fahrenheit.
Line 12 muffin cups with cupcake papers.

Beat the 2 egg whites with a whisk for a couple of
seconds and combine with the 1 cup of apples
(chopped), 3/4 cup of milk, 1/4 cup of canola oil, and 1/4
cup of honey in a bowl. In a separate bowl, combine the
2 cups of whole wheat flour, 1 tablespoon of baking
powder, 1 teaspoon of cinnamon (ground), and 1/2
teaspoon of salt. Mix the dry ingredients in with the wet
ingredients until just moistened. Batter will be lumpy.
Spoon equal amounts into the 12 cupcake paper lined
muffin cups and bake until the top turns a golden
brown, about 20 minutes.

Buttermilk Fruit Nut Muffins

These muffins taste great with bananas, walnuts and blueberries. Makes 1 dozen muffins.

What You'll Need:

1 banana (ripe, mashed)
1 egg
1 1/2 cups of wheat bran
1 cup of buttermilk
3/4 cup of blueberries
3/4 cup of whole wheat flour
2/3 cup of brown sugar (packed)
1/2 cup of oat bran
1/2 cup of walnuts (chopped)
1/3 cup of canola oil
1 teaspoon of baking powder
1 teaspoon of baking soda
1/2 teaspoon of vanilla extract

How to Make It:

Prep: Preheat the oven to 400 degrees Fahrenheit. Line 12 muffin cups with cupcake papers.

Combine the 1 1/2 cups of wheat bran and 1 cup of

buttermilk in a bowl. In a separate bowl, combine the egg (beat with a whisk first) with the 1 banana (ripe, mashed), 2/3 cup of brown sugar (packed), 1/3 cup of canola oil, and 1/2 teaspoon of vanilla extract. In yet another bowl, combine the 3/4 cup of whole wheat flour, 1/2 cup of oat bran, 1 teaspoon of baking powder, and 1 teaspoon of baking soda. Combine the dry ingredients with the wet ingredients (all 3 bowls). Fold in the 3/4 cup of blueberries and the 1/2 cup of walnuts (chopped). Evenly fill each of the lined muffin cups and bake for 20 minutes in the hot oven.

California Blueberry Smoothie

Have a bit of California with the addition of avocados in this delicious breakfast smoothie. Makes 2 servings.

What You'll Need:

2 containers of yogurt (6 oz. each, Greek, plain)
1/2 of an avocado (peeled, pitted, chunked)
2 cups of blueberries (frozen)
1 cup of almond milk
1 cup of water
1/4 cup of ice

How to Make It:

Combine 2 containers of yogurt (6 oz. each, Greek, plain), 1/2 of an avocado (peeled, pitted, chunked), 2 cups of blueberries (frozen), 1 cup of almond milk, 1 cup of water, and 1/4 cup of ice in a blender or food processor and blend until smooth. Pour into 2 tall glasses.

Honey Bran Muffins

These whole grain muffins give you a great start to the day. Makes a dozen muffins.

What You'll Need:

2 eggs
2 3/4 cups of wheat bran
1 1/4 cups of milk
1 cup of flour (whole wheat)
1 cup of raisins
1 cup of wheat germ
1 cup of yogurt (plain)
2/3 cup of honey
2/3 cup of oat bran
3 tablespoons of canola oil
1 tablespoon of barley malt flour
2 teaspoons of baking powder
2 teaspoons of baking soda
2 teaspoons of ginger (ground)

How to Make It:

Prep: Preheat the oven to 350 degrees Fahrenheit. Line 12 muffin cups with cupcake papers.

Combine the 2 3/4 cups of wheat bran, 1 cup of flour (whole wheat), 1 cup of wheat germ, 2/3 cup of oat bran, 1 tablespoon of barley malt flour, 2 teaspoons of baking powder, 2 teaspoons of baking soda, and 2 teaspoons of ginger (ground). In a separate bowl combine the 2 eggs and beat with a whisk then add the 1 1/4 cups of milk, 1 cup of yogurt (plain), 2/3 cup of honey, and 3 tablespoons of canola oil. Stir in the dry ingredients until barely combined. Fold in the cup of raisins. Equally, spoon the batter into the 12 lined muffin cups. Bake in the hot oven until golden brown and an inserted toothpick in the middle comes out clean, about 25 minutes.

Hot Quinoa Breakfast Cereal

A delicious bowl of hot quinoa cereal with apples and cinnamon help to start the morning right. Makes 2 servings.

What You'll Need:

2 apples (small, Granny Smith, peeled, cored, chopped)
2/3 cup of apple juice
2/3 cup of quinoa
2/3 cup of water
2 teaspoons of honey
2 teaspoons of cinnamon

How to Make It:

Combine the 2/3 cup of apple juice, 2/3 cup of quinoa, and 2/3 cup of water in a saucepan and turn heat to high to bring to a boil. Turn to medium low and add the 2 teaspoons of cinnamon and stir while cooking for another 10 minutes. Add the 2 apples (small, Granny Smith, peeled, cored, chopped) and continue cooking for 10 more minutes. Split between 2 bowls and add a teaspoon of honey to each bowl, stir and eat.

Loose Granola

This is the perfect granola to eat however you want, in a bowl with your fingers, as a topping on yogurt or ice cream or in bowl with your favorite milk and a spoon. Makes 12 servings.

What You'll Need:

2 1/2 cups of oats (rolled)
1 cup of almonds (slivered, toasted)
1 cup of coconut flakes
1/2 cup of honey
1/2 cup of raisins
1/4 cup of canola oil
3/4 teaspoon of cinnamon (ground)

How to Make It:

Combine the 2 1/2 cups of oats (rolled), 1 cup of almonds (slivered, toasted), 1 cup of coconut flakes, 1/2 cup of raisins, and 3/4 teaspoon of cinnamon (ground) in a bowl. Combine the 1/2 cup of honey with the 1/4 cup of canola oil, drizzle over the top of the oat mixture, and toss to combine. Spread onto the prepared baking sheet and bake for half an hour, stirring every 10 minutes. Loosen the granola upon removal from the oven, and then set aside to cool completely. Break apart and store in an airtight container at room temperature.

Oatmeal Nut Bars

This is a delicious breakfast bar that is packed full of goodness from oats, apples and walnuts. Makes 36 bars.

What You'll Need:

2 1/2 cups of oats (rolled)
1 cup of brown sugar (packed)
1 cup of flour (all-purpose)
1 cup of walnuts (chopped)
1/2 cup of butter (softened)
1/4 cup of applesauce
2 teaspoons of cinnamon (ground)
1 teaspoon of vanilla extract

How to Make It:

Prep: Preheat the oven to 350 degrees Fahrenheit. Spray a 9x13 inch baking pan with cooking spray.

Combine the 1 cup of brown sugar (packed) and the 1/2 cup of butter (softened) in a bowl. Add the 2 1/2 cups of oats (rolled), 1 cup of flour (all-purpose), 2 teaspoons of cinnamon (ground), and 1 teaspoon of vanilla extract and mix well. Add the 1 cup of walnuts (chopped) and

1/4 cup of applesauce and combine. Put the batter into the prepared 9x13 pan and bake in the hot oven until golden brown about 35 minutes. Cool completely and cut into 36 squares.

Oatmeal with Cinnamon Apples

A hearty bowl of oatmeal starts the day right. Makes 2 servings.

What You'll Need:

1 apple (cored, chopped, peeled)
1 cup of milk
1 cup of water
2/3 cup of oats (rolled)
1/4 cup of apple juice
2 teaspoons of honey
1 teaspoon of cinnamon (ground)

How to Make It:

Combine the 1 apple (cored, chopped, peeled), 1 cup of water, and 1/4 cup of apple juice in a saucepan with heat turned to high. Bring to a boil and add the 2/3 cup of oats (rolled) and the 1 teaspoon of cinnamon (ground) and stir. Bring to a second boil and turn the heat to low and cook for 3 minutes, stirring often. Spoon into 2 bowls and add a teaspoon of honey to each bowl, stir and eat.

Peach Berry Smoothie

This is a delicious peach dominate smoothie with the refreshing addition of blueberries, strawberries, and blackberries. Makes 2 servings.

What You'll Need:

1 can of peaches (sliced, drained)
1/2 cup of blackberries
1/2 cup of blueberries
1/2 cup of strawberries
1/4 cup of ice
2 tablespoons of honey

How to Make It:

Combine 1 can of peaches (sliced, drained), 1/2 cup of blackberries, 1/2 cup of blueberries, 1/2 cup of strawberries, 1/4 cup of ice, and 2 tablespoons of honey in a blender or food processor and blend until smooth. Pour into 2 tall glasses.

Peanut Butter Muffins

This is a different twist to the breakfast muffin. Try it with a dollop of your favorite natural jam. Makes 1 dozen muffins.

What You'll Need:

1 egg
1 1/4 cups of milk
1/4 cup of flour (all purpose)
3/4 cup of brown sugar
3/4 cups of oats (rolled)
1/4 cup of peanut butter (natural)
1 tablespoon of baking powder
1/2 teaspoon of salt

How to Make It:

Prep: Preheat the oven to 375 degrees Fahrenheit. Add cupcake papers to 12 muffin cups.

Combine the 1/4 cup of flour (all purpose), 3/4 cup of brown sugar, 3/4 cups of oats (rolled), 1 tablespoon of baking powder, and 1/2 teaspoon of salt. In a separate bowl beat the egg with a whisk then combine with the 1 1/4 cups of milk and 1/4 cup of peanut butter (natural).

Blend the dry ingredients into the wet ingredients. Divide the batter into the 12 lined muffin cups. Bake in the hot oven for 17 minutes or until a toothpick inserted in the middle comes out clean.

Pumpkin Apple Smoothie

Combine apples with pumpkin and sprinkle in the right seasonings and you have this delicious breakfast smoothie. Makes 2 servings.

What You'll Need:

2 containers of yogurt (6 oz. each, vanilla)
1 banana (peeled, frozen, chopped)
2 cups of apple juice
1/2 cup of pumpkin pie filling
1/4 cup of ice
1 teaspoon of cinnamon (ground)
Nutmeg (ground)

How to Make It:

Combine the 2 containers of yogurt (6 oz. each, vanilla), 1 banana (peeled, frozen, chopped), 2 cups of apple juice, 1/2 cup of pumpkin pie filling, 1/4 cup of ice, 1 teaspoon of cinnamon (ground), and a couple of dashes of ground nutmeg in a blender or food processor and blend until smooth. Pour into 2 tall glasses.

Desserts and Snacks

Roasted Nuts

Servings: varies

Ingredients:

1 cup raw walnut halves
½ cup raw whole almonds
½ cup raw whole macadamia nuts
¼ cup raw pumpkin seeds
2 tbsp pineapple juice
1 tbsp brown sugar
1 tsp walnut oil
½ tsp cinnamon
½ tsp nutmeg
a pinch of salt

Preparation:

Preheat your oven to 325 F. While the oven is heating, combine all of your ingredients in a large bowl and stir to combine. Spread the mixture on a baking sheet and bake for about 30 minutes or until the nuts are roasted and sticky, stirring every 10 minutes. Serve warm or allow them to cool – these can also be stored in an airtight container for up to 1 week at room temperature.

Granola Bars with Fruit

Number of servings: 16

Ingredients:

1 ¼ cup rolled oats
2/3 cup dried cranberries or blueberries, chopped
¼ cup pecans or walnuts, chopped
1 cup brown sugar
1 egg
1 egg white
1 tbsp all purpose flour
1 tbsp vegetable oil
1 tsp cinnamon
1 tsp vanilla extract
a pinch of salt

Preparation:

Preheat the oven to 350 F. Once the oven is hot, spread
the rolled oats on a baking sheet and bake for 15 – 20
minutes, stirring occasionally – the oats will become
fragrant and lightly browned. Remove from the oven
and set aside.

Reduce the heat to 325 F and lightly oil a 8" x 11" baking

pan. Whisk together the egg, egg white, vegetable oil, brown sugar, vanilla extract and salt in a large bowl until combined. Mix in the toasted oats, dried fruit, nuts and all purpose flour. Spread the mixture in the baking sheet and bake for about 35 minutes or until the mixture turns golden brown. Remove from the oven and allow to cool before cutting into 16 bars (using a lightly oiled knife will make this process much easier).

Blueberry Shortbread Bars

Number of servings: 18

Ingredients:

The filling:
3 pints fresh blueberries
½ cup sugar
3 tbsp corn starch
The crust:
2 ½ cups all purpose flour
1 cup butter, softened at room temperature
2/3 cup powdered sugar
1 tsp vanilla extract
The topping:
2/3 cup rolled oats
½ cup all purpose flour
1/3 cup brown sugar
1 tsp cinnamon
½ cup butter

Preparation:

Preheat your oven to 375 F. Beat the softened butter, powdered sugar and vanilla extract together until the mixture is light and fluffy. Beat in the flour until just combined. Transfer the dough to a large (9" x 13") baking pan or jelly roll pan and press it firmly onto the bottom of the pan to form a crust. Bake the crust for 20 minutes, or until it becomes golden brown. Remove from oven and allow it to cool slightly.

While the crust is in the oven, make your filling. Add the blueberries, sugar, cornstarch, blueberries and a little water (about 2 tbsp) to a saucepan and bring to a boil, stirring often to dissolve the sugar and corn starch. Boil for 1 – 2 minutes and remove from heat.

You can now make your streusel topping as well. In a large bowl, mix together the rolled oats, flour, brown sugar and cinnamon. Cut the butter into the dry ingredients until it reaches the consistency of coarse bread crumbs.

Spread the blueberry filling evenly over the crust once it has cooled. Top with the streusel and return to the oven for 35 – 40 minutes, or until the streusel is lightly browned. Remove from the oven and place the pan on a wire rack to cool to room temperature before slicing and serving.

Blueberry, Chocolate and Walnut Parfait

Number of servings: 4

Ingredients:

½ cup blueberries (fresh or frozen and thawed)
2 cups plain Greek yogurt
2 tbsp miniature dark chocolate chips
½ cup granola
chopped walnuts

Preparation:

Place 1 tbsp of blueberries at the bottom of 4 parfait glasses, followed by ¼ cup Greek yogurt. The next layer is 1 tsp chocolate chips, 1 tsp granola and a few walnut pieces. Repeat the process to form a second layer. Serve immediately or chill in the refrigerator until you're ready to serve.

Dark Chocolate Cake

Number of servings: 8

Ingredients:

1¾ cups pastry flour (use whole wheat pastry flour if you have it)
1 ½ cups dark chocolate (either dark chocolate chips or bars broken into small pieces)
¾ cup milk (soy milk or almond milk may be substituted if desired)
½ cup apple juice or apple cider
½ cup maple syrup
¼ cup canola oil
2 ½ tbsp flax seeds
1 tbsp baking powder
2 tsp vanilla extract
¼ tsp salt

Preparation:

Start by preheating your oven to 350 F. Oil a 9" cake pan. In a large mixing bowl, combine the pastry flour, salt and baking powder; mix well and set aside. Grind the flax seeds in a blender or coffee grinder until they're powdered. Add the oil, apple juice or cider, vanilla extract and maple syrup to the blender and blend until thoroughly combined.

In a saucepan, heat the milk (or soy or almond milk) and chocolate over low heat for about 4 minutes or until the chocolate is melted. Add the chocolate mixture and the flax seed mixture to the dry ingredients and mix well until a smooth batter is formed.

Pour your batter into the cake pan and bake for 40 – 45 minutes; you'll be able to tell the cake is done when a toothpick inserted in the center of the cake comes out clean. Remove the cake from the oven and allow it to cool for at least half an hour before removing from the pan. Serve either plain or frosted, if desired.

Superfoods Cookbook Conclusion

Eating healthy doesn't have to mean not eating food that tastes good – or even giving up the foods that you like! There are almost limitless ways to work in the superfoods which are the stars of the recipes in this book into your diet. No matter what your dietary preferences happen to be (unless you've been eating nothing but heavily processed foods of course and even then, the recipes here have hopefully shown you a better and tastier way to eat), you can eat a diet rich in superfoods and reap their nutritional benefits.

The fact is that many of the healthiest foods also happen to be absolutely delicious. If there is a secret to making eating healthy as delicious as the recipes here show that it really can be, it's this: use high quality, healthy ingredients and allow their flavors to shine through. Even if you never thought that you liked, say, kale, you may find yourself a fan once you've tried it in many of these recipes.

Try cooking your way through this superfoods cookbook and you'll soon discover a whole new way of eating –

one which gives you a stronger immune system, better health and generally helps you to feel (and maybe even look) younger and healthier than you have in a long time, or perhaps ever. Feel free to use these recipes as a source of inspiration for your own culinary experiments as well. You may find that you can find many new ways to enjoy superfoods at your table and start getting the nutrition that your body needs not from nutritional supplements, but from where you should be naturally: from your diet.

19698095R00078

Printed in Great Britain
by Amazon